FROM BIRTH TO FIVE YEARS
Children's Developmental Progress

Mary D. Sheridan

Revised and updated by

Marion Frost and **Dr Ajay Sharma**

First published by The NFER Publishing Company 1973.
Second impression 1974
Third and expanded edition 1975
Fourth impression 1976
Fifth impression 1977
Sixth impression 1978
Seventh impression 1980

Reprinted by the NFER-Nelson Publishing Company Ltd,
1981, 1982, 1983, 1984, 1985, 1986, 1987, 1988 (twice), 1989, 1990, 1991

Reprinted in 1992 (twice), 1993, 1994 (twice), 1995 by Routledge, 11 Fetter Lane, London
EC4P 4EE

This revised and updated edition first published in Great Britain 1997 by Routledge Ltd.

Published under licence in Australia by the Australian Council for Educational Research 1988.
Reprinted 1990, 1993, 1994, 1996, 1999, 2000, 2001, 2002, 2003, 2005, 2006, 2007, 2008

This edition published under licence in 1998 (in paperback only) by ACER Press
19 Prospect Hill Road, Camberwell, Melbourne, Victoria 3124, Australia

Printed by BPA Print Group.

National Library of Australia
Cataloguing-in-Publication data:

Sheridan, Mary D. (Mary Dorothy).

From birth to five years: children's developmental progress.

ISBN 0 86431 269 5

1. Child development. 2. Infants - Development. I. Sharma, Ajay. II. Frost, Marion. III. Australian
Council for Educational Research. IV. Title.

155.422

Illustrations by Oxford Illustrators

Cover photography by Lupe Cunha

Contents

Acknowledgements

The original version of the developmental charts used in this book came from the investigative work carried out by Mary D. Sheridan, and first appeared in the publication entitled *The Developmental Progress of Infants and Young Children* (HMSO 1960) with second and third editions published in 1968 and 1975.

The editors of this current edition would like to thank all those people who gave invaluable assistance during the production of this book, in particular the following: Auriol Drew, Speech and Language Therapist; Dorothy Duffy, Specialist Health Visitor for Children with Special Needs; Sally French, Senior Lecturer; Marie Louise Irvine, Eva and Nicky; and Gloria Lowe, Kwame and Yohannes.

Introduction

From Birth to Five Years is designed as a source of information and reference for all professionals and students who wish to increase their knowledge of the developmental progress of infants and young children. This may include health visitors, general practitioners, paediatricians, child therapists, paediatric nurse trainees, nursery nurses and those studying for vocational qualifications in child care. It is essential that all who work with young children appreciate the range of normal development in order to facilitate the identification of developmental differences.

The previous edition of this book was based on research carried out by Mary D. Sheridan, which was concerned with discovering appropriate testing procedures to aid paediatric diagnosis, improve the clinical management of children with developmental disorders and provide guidance for parents and teachers (Sheridan 1975). While continuing to recognise the importance of detecting disorders and providing effective support for children with special needs related to developmental differences, the current philosophy of a child health promotion programme places greater emphasis on preventive health care. The prevention of ill health and the promotion of health require a change in the professional–client relationship, with the recognition that parents should be regarded as equal partners in the care and management of their children. This book, therefore, has been revised and updated to take account of these changes and to give information based on what is currently accepted as best practice.

The main section, Section 1, retains much of the work of Mary D. Sheridan and consists of illustrated charts of developmental progress, sequenced in chronological order and spanning the period of childhood from birth to five years of age. The charts are divided into four key areas:

- Posture and large movements
- Vision and fine movements
- Hearing and speech
- Social behaviour and play

The identification of these areas assists the understanding of the variance between ages at which children achieve developmental skills, although the influence of heredity, and social and environmental factors, must also be taken into account. The charts should be used to recognise both the *abilities* and the *needs* of children in relation to developmental differences. It is characteristic of many children, and particularly those with special needs, that the profile of development will be uneven across the different areas. Understanding the process of child development is necessary for promoting healthy development and for identifying areas where further investigation is required.

The second section of this book deals with patterns of development which are significant for the understanding of developmental differences. Variations in the development of posture and movement, vision, hearing, communication, language and speech are detailed, and advice is given as to when referrals for specialist examination should be considered. Age-appropriate checks for identifying hearing and vision disorders have been included and acknowledge the importance of seeking out parental concerns. It is crucial to detect disorders as early as possible if effective interventions to prevent or reduce impairment are to be implemented.

The third section provides an index of support services for parents and carers of young children with special needs. Raising parents' and carers' awareness of the available support for their child can play a vital part in reducing the impact of disability as well as aiding the adjustment to disorders where there is little or no chance of improvement.

Although, as Illingworth (1992) suggests, it is frequently difficult to distinguish between normal and abnormal development, early detection of disorders is vital for both children and their families. There is no doubt that the younger the age at which children with physical, intellectual, emotional or social disabilities are identified, the more likely it is that appropriate interventions can be planned to enable them to develop to their individual potential. Children with developmental needs should be encouraged to be as independent as possible, so that participation in everyday life can be achieved.

The United Nations Convention on the Rights of the Child states that children are a vulnerable group in society and proposes that all children should enjoy the highest attainable standard of care, while recognising that those with special needs require particular care. It is, therefore, essential that all those who work with young children are familiar with the sequences and patterns of developmental progress and appropriate interventions for identifying and supporting those with special needs. This edition of *From Birth to Five Years* is intended to provide such information and thus will continue to be a useful aid in promoting the health of children.

T his section considers the developmental progress of children from birth to five years of age. The information is not intended to be a checklist against which development can be measured, but provides an outline of the usual developmental progress for the specified age groups. There is a great deal of variation in the age at which different children achieve the same skill, and a few may miss out some developmental activities such as crawling. Minor variations are not usually considered a cause for concern, although, as a general rule, the younger the child the more significant is the variation. It must be remembered that infants and children will also function at differing levels depending on such factors as their physical or emotional state of health. The following charts should, therefore, be viewed as guidelines for studying the developmental progress of young children. Professionals and students can use them to look ahead at the expected developmental sequences, utilising the information to facilitate a child's development.

Illustrated Charts

of Children's

Developmental

Progress

THE NEWBORN BABY

During the first few days of life there is a great variability in the behaviour of babies depending not only upon the baby's maturity and physical condition, but also upon its state of alertness or drowsiness, hunger or satiation. Sensitive support for the mother is required, including help in establishing breast feeding. An examination of the newborn baby must include a discussion with the parents regarding any concerns about the normal behaviour of newborn babies, and findings must be communicated in a manner that is comprehensible to the parents. The following description will help in understanding the range of behaviour expected from a newborn baby.

The states of sleep and wakefulness

The first few days of a baby's life are usually composed of long periods of sleep interspersed with short periods when the baby is awake. The duration of wakefulness lengthens gradually and includes periods of fretfulness, crying and calmness. The responsiveness of the baby depends on the state of sleep or wakefulness. From the first days of life the infant establishes interaction with his or her parent by changing states of wakefulness (Brazelton 1995). Any examination of the newborn should be carried out in the optimal state of wakefulness, when the infant is quiet with eyes open and with or without irregular movements of arms and legs (Prechtl 1977).

Posture and large movements

At birth the arms and legs are characteristically stiff (hypertonia) and the trunk and neck floppy (hypotonia). Held in ventral suspension, the head drops below the plane of the body and the arms and legs are kept partly flexed. Pulled to sitting, marked head lag is present. Held in a sitting position the back is curved and the head falls forward. Placed on the abdomen (prone) the head is promptly turned sideways. The buttocks are humped up with the knees tucked under the abdomen. The arms are close to the chest with the elbows fully flexed. Lying on the back (supine), the arms and legs are kept semi-flexed and the posture is symmetrical. Babies born after breech presentation usually keep their legs extended.

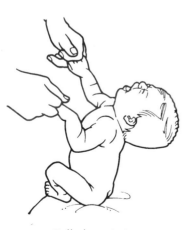

Pulled to sitting

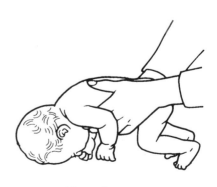

Ventral suspension

These represent neurological maturation of the newborn and are present from the gestational age of thirty-two weeks. Some reflexes may help in establishing symmetry of movement, but others are of limited value in the examination of a full-term newborn infant. The Moro reflex is the best known of all the neonatal reflexes. It can be produced in several ways. The usual method is by sudden, slight (2.5 cm) dropping of the examiner's hand supporting the baby's head. The response consists of symmetrical wide abduction of the arms and opening of the hands. Within moments the arms come together again simulating an embrace. The reflex fades rapidly and is not normally present after six months of age.

Reflex standing and reflex walking are apparent during the early weeks of life if the feet are placed on a firm surface.

Reflex rooting and sucking behaviour is apparent during feeding times. Strong and symmetrical palmar grasp reflex is present, but fades rapidly over the next four to five months.

Babies are sensitive to light and sound at birth. Visual responsiveness varies at birth. From birth onwards, or within a few days, infants turn their eyes towards a large and diffuse source of light, and close their eyes to sudden bright light. Infants cannot accommodate until the age of three months, and an object or face must be brought to a distance of thirty centimetres to obtain interest and fixation. Infants usually turn their eyes to follow a face moved slowly within a quarter circle.

The startle reaction to sudden loud sounds is present. Eyes may be turned towards a nearby source of continued sound, such as a voiced 'ah-ah' or a bell. Momentary stilling to weaker continuous sounds is also seen.

Within a few days of birth, infants establish an interaction with their carers through eye contact, spontaneous or imitative facial gestures and modulation of their sleep–wakefulness state. Interactions and other subtle indications of individuality shown by babies from birth onwards strengthen the emotional ties between the infant and its carers.

The primary reflexes

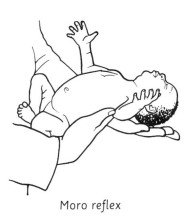

Moro reflex

Hearing and vision

Social interaction and the formation of attachments

AGE 1 MONTH

Posture and large movements

Lying on back (supine), keeps head to one side with arm and leg on face side outstretched, or both arms flexed; knees apart, soles of feet turned inwards.

Large, jerky movements of limbs, arms more active than legs. At rest, keeps hands closed and thumbs turned in, but beginning to open hands from time to time. Fingers and toes fan out during extensor movements of limbs.

When cheek touched at corner of mouth, turns to same side in attempt to suck finger. When ear gently rubbed, turns head away.

When lifted from cot, head falls loosely unless supported. Pulled to sit, head lags until body vertical when head is held momentarily erect before falling forwards. Held sitting, back is one complete curve.

In ventral suspension, head in line with body and hips semi-extended.

Placed on abdomen (prone), head immediately turns to side; arms and legs flexed, elbows away from body, buttocks moderately high.

Held standing on hard surface, presses down feet, straightens body and usually makes a reflex forward 'walking' movement. Stimulation of dorsum of foot against table edge produces 'stepping up over curb'.

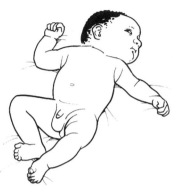

Lying on back (supine)

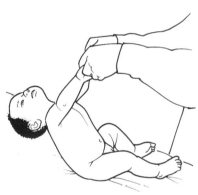

Pulled to sit

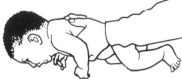

Held in ventral suspension

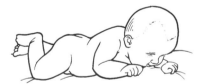

Placed on abdomen (prone)

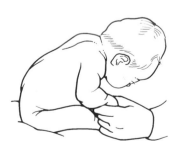

Held sitting

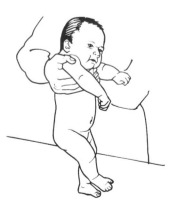

Reflex 'walking' movement

Pupils react to light. Turns head and eyes towards diffuse light source – stares at diffuse brightness of window, table lamp or lightly coloured blank wall.

Follows pencil light briefly with eyes, at a distance of thirty centimetres. Shuts eyes tightly when pencil light shone directly into them.

Gaze caught and held by dangling bright toy gently moved in line of vision at fifteen to twenty-five centimetres, towards and away from face. Focuses and follows with eyes slow movements of face or object from side towards midline horizontally with face through quarter circle or more, before head falls back to side. From about three weeks, watches familiar nearby face when being fed or talked to with increasingly alert facial expression.

Defensive blink present by six to eight weeks.

AGE 1 MONTH

Vision and fine movements

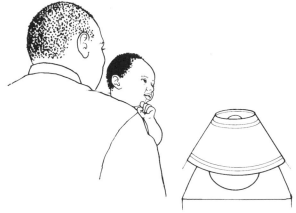

Turns to diffuse light source

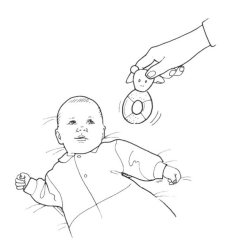

Gazes at toy moved towards and away from face

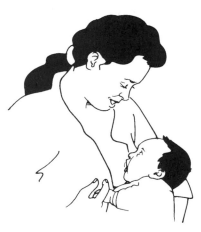

Regards familiar face when being fed

5

AGE 1 MONTH

Hearing and speech

Startled by sudden noises, stiffens, quivers, blinks, screws up eyes, extends limbs, fans out fingers and toes and may cry. Movements momentarily 'frozen' when small bell rung gently; may move eyes and head towards sound source, but cannot yet localise sound.

Stops whimpering; and usually turns towards sound of nearby soothing human voice or loud and prolonged noise, e.g. vacuum cleaner, but not when screaming or feeding. Utters little guttural noises when content. Coos responsively to parent's or carer's talk from about five or six weeks.

Cries lustily when hungry or uncomfortable.

Note: Babies with hearing impairment also cry and vocalise in this reflex fashion but when very severely impaired do not usually show startle reflex to sudden noise. Babies with severe visual impairment may also move eyes towards a sound-making instrument. Visual following and auditory response must therefore always be tested separately.

Social behaviour and play

Sucks well. Sleeps most of the time when not being fed or handled.

Expression still vague but becoming more alert later, progressing to social smile and responsive vocalisations at about five or six weeks.

Hands normally closed, but if opened, grasps finger when palm is touched.

Stops crying when picked up and spoken to. Turns to regard nearby speaker's face.

Needs support to head when being carried, dressed and bathed.

Passive acceptance of bath and dressing routines gradually gives way to incipient awareness and response.

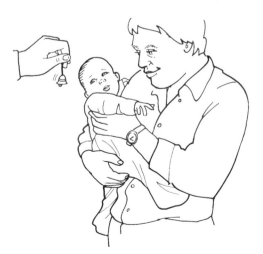

Stops whimpering to listen to sudden noise

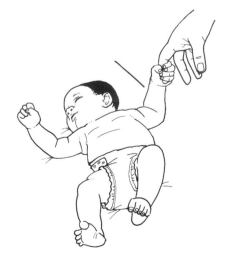

Grasps finger

Lying on back, prefers to lie with head in midline. Limbs more pliable, movements smoother and more continuous. Waves arms symmetrically. Hands loosely open.

Brings hands together from sides into midline over chest or chin. Kicks vigorously, legs alternating or occasionally together.

When pulled to sit, little or no head lag. Held sitting, back is straight except in lumbar region. Head held erect and steady for several seconds before bobbing forwards.

In ventral suspension, head held well above line of body, hips and shoulders extended.

Lying on abdomen, lifts head and upper chest well up in midline, using forearms to support and often actively scratching at surface with hands, with buttocks flat.

Held standing with feet on hard surface, sags at knees.

AGE 3 MONTHS

Posture and large movements

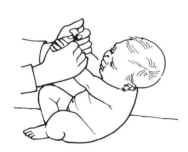

Pulled to sit

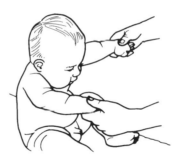

Held sitting, lumbar curve

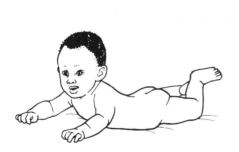

Lying on abdomen

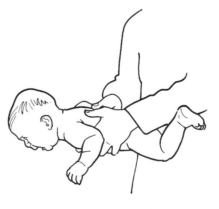

Ventral suspension

AGE 3 MONTHS

Vision and fine movements

Visually very alert, particularly preoccupied by nearby human face. Moves head deliberately to gaze attentively around. Follows adult's movements within available visual field.

Follows dangling toy at fifteen to twenty-five centimetres from face through half circle horizontally from side to side and usually also vertically from chest to brow.

Hand regard when lying supine – watches movement of own hands before face and engages in finger play. Beginning to clasp and unclasp hands, pressing palms of hands together.

Eager anticipation of breast or bottle feed.

Regards small still objects within fifteen to twenty-five centimetres for more than a second or two, but seldom fixates continuously. Converges eyes as dangling toy is moved towards face. Defensive blink is clearly shown.

Holds rattle for a few moments when placed in hand, may move towards face – sometimes bashing chin – but seldom capable of regarding it at the same time until sixteen to eighteen weeks of age.

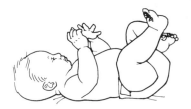

Hand regard and finger play

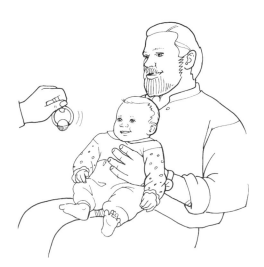

Follows dangling toy

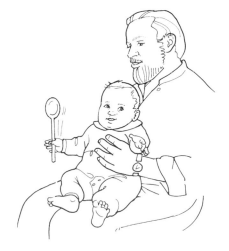

Holds toy but cannot yet coordinate hands and eyes

Hearing and speech

Sudden loud noises still distress, provoking blinking, screwing up of eyes, crying and turning away. Definite quieting or smiling to sound of familiar voice before being touched, but not when screaming. Vocalises delightedly when spoken to or pleased; also when alone. Cries when uncomfortable or annoyed. Quietens to sound of rattle or small bell rung gently out of sight.

Turns eyes and/or head towards sound source, e.g. nearby voice; brows may wrinkle and eyes dilate. May move head from side to side as if searching for sound source.

Often sucks or licks lips in response to sounds of preparation for feeding.

Shows excitement at sound of approaching voices, footsteps, running bathwater, etc.

Note: Babies with severe hearing impairment may be obviously startled by carer's appearance beside cot.

AGE 3 MONTHS

Hearing and speech

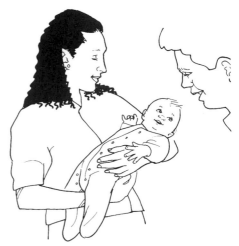

Turns to nearby voice

Fixes eyes unblinkingly on parent's or carer's face when feeding, with contented purposeful gaze.

Beginning to react to familiar situations, shown by smiles, coos and excited movements, recognition of the preparations for feeds, baths, etc. Now definitely enjoys bathing and caring routines.

Responds with obvious pleasure to friendly handling, especially when accompanied by playful tickling and vocal sounds.

Needs support at shoulders when being bathed and dressed.

Social behaviour and play

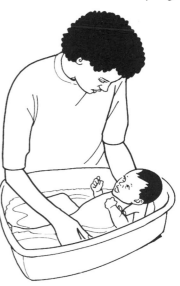

Responds with pleasure to friendly handling

Enjoys bath

AGE 6 MONTHS

Posture and large movements

Lying on back, raises head to look at feet. Lifts legs into vertical position and grasps one foot, and then later two feet.

Sits with support and turns head from side to side to look around. Moves arms in brisk, purposeful fashion and holds them up to be lifted. When hands grasped, braces shoulders and pulls self to sitting.

Kicks strongly, legs alternating. Can roll over from front to back and usually from back to front.

Held sitting, head is firmly erect and back straight.

Placed on abdomen, lifts head and chest well up, supporting self on extended arms and flattened palms.

Held standing with feet touching hard surface, bears weight on feet and bounces up and down actively.

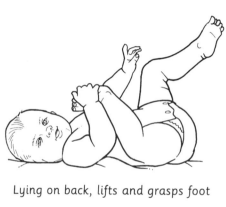

Lying on back, lifts and grasps foot

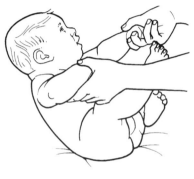

Pulls self to sitting, braces shoulders

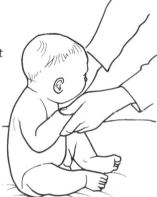

Held sitting, back straight

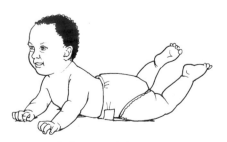

Lying on abdomen, arms extended

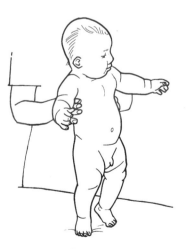

Held standing, takes weight on legs

Visually insatiable: moves head and eyes eagerly in every direction when attention is distracted. Follows adult's or child's activities across room with purposeful alertness.

Eyes move in unison: any squint now definitely abnormal.

Immediately stares at interesting small objects or toys within fifteen to thirty centimetres and, almost simultaneously, stretches out both hands to grasp. Uses whole hand to palmar grasp and passes toy from one hand to another.

When toy falls from hand within visual field, watches to resting place. When toy falls outside visual field, searches vaguely around with eyes and hands, or forgets it.

AGE 6 MONTHS

Vision and fine movements

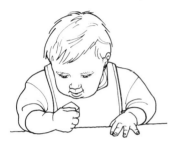

Palmar grasp

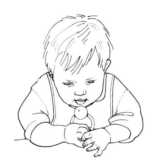

Grasps toy with both hands

Turns immediately to a familiar voice across the room. Listens to voice even if adult not in view. Vocalises tunefully to self and others, using sing-song vowel sounds or single and double syllables, e.g. 'a-a', 'muh', 'goo', 'der', 'adah', 'er-leh', 'aroo'.

Laughs, chuckles and squeals aloud in play. Screams with annoyance.

Shows evidence of selective response to different emotional tones of familiar voice.

Turns to source when hears sounds at ear level.

Hearing and speech

AGE 6 MONTHS

Social behaviour and play

Uses hands competently to reach for and grasp small toys. Mainly uses two-handed scooping-in approach, but will occasionally use a single hand.

Takes everything to mouth.

Finds feet as well as hands interesting to move about and regard: sometimes uses feet to help in grasping objects.

Places hand on breast while feeding; or, if fed with formula milk, puts hand on bottle and pats it. May attempt to grasp cup if used.

When offered a rattle, reaches for it immediately and shakes deliberately to make a sound, often regarding it closely at the same time. Manipulates objects attentively, passing them frequently from hand to hand.

Shows delighted response to active play.

Still friendly with strangers but occasionally shows some shyness or even slight anxiety when approached too nearly or abruptly, especially if familiar adult is out of sight.

Note: Becomes more reserved with strangers from about seven months.

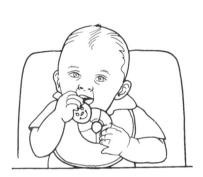

Takes everything to mouth

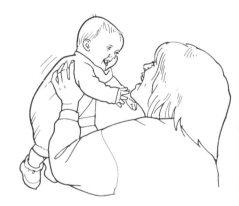

Delighted response to active play

Sits unsupported on the floor and can lean forward to pick up a toy without losing balance, and sits and manipulates toys. Can turn body to look sideways while stretching out to pick up toy from floor.

Progresses on floor by rolling, wriggling on abdomen or crawling.

Pulls to standing, holding on to support for a few moments, but cannot lower self. Falls backwards with a bump.

Held standing, steps purposefully on alternate feet.

AGE 9 MONTHS

Posture and large movements

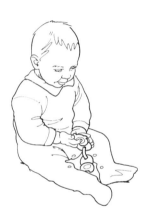

Sits on floor and manipulates toys

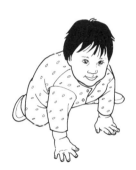

Attempts to crawl

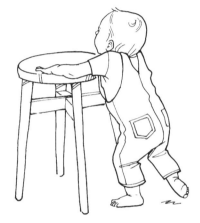

Pulls to standing

AGE 9 MONTHS

Vision and fine movements

Visually very attentive to people, objects and happenings in the environment. Immediately stretches out to grasp a small toy when offered, with one hand leading. Manipulates toy with a lively interest, passing from hand to hand and turning over. Regards unoffered but accessible toy before grasping, especially if unfamiliar.

Pokes at small object with index finger and begins to point at more distant object with same finger.

Grasps string between finger and thumb in scissor fashion in order to pull toy towards self. Picks up small object between finger and thumb with 'inferior' pincer grasp.

Can release toy from grasp by dropping or pressing against a firm surface, but cannot yet place down voluntarily.

Looks in correct direction for falling or fallen toys. Watches activities of people or animals within three or four metres with sustained interest for several minutes.

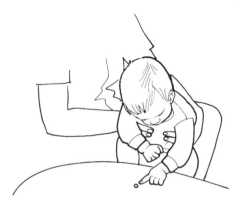

Pokes at small objects using index finger

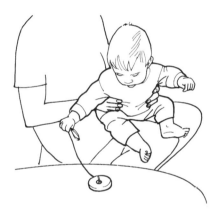

Grasps string in scissor fashion

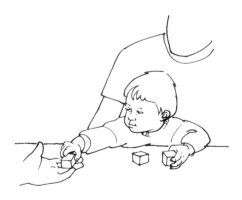

Lifts cube, but cannot put down voluntarily

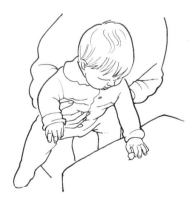

Picks up small object with pincer grasp

Eagerly attentive to everyday sounds, particularly voice.

Vocalises deliberately as a means of inter-personal communication in friendliness or annoyance. Shouts to attract attention, listens, then shouts again.

Babbles loudly and tunefully in long repetitive strings of syllables, e.g. 'dad-dad', 'mam-mam', 'adaba', 'agaga'. Babble is practised largely for self-amusement, but also as a sign of favoured communication.

Understands 'no' and 'bye-bye'.

Imitates playful vocal and other sounds, e.g. smacking lips, cough, 'brrr'.

Turns to search and localise faint sounds on either side.

Note: The vocalisations of children with severely impaired hearing remain at the primitive level and do not usually progress to repetitive tuneful babble. Poor or monotonous vocalisations after eight or nine months of age should always arouse suspicion.

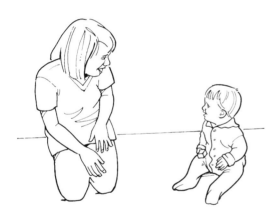

Attentive to voice of familiar person

AGE 9 MONTHS

Social behaviour and play

Holds, bites and chews a small piece of food. Puts hands on breast or around bottle or cup when drinking. Tries to grasp spoon when being fed.

Throws body back and stiffens in annoyance or resistance, usually protesting vocally at same time.

Clearly distinguishes strangers from familiars and requires reassurance before accepting their advances; clings to known person and hides face.

Still takes everything to mouth.

Grasps bell by handle and rings in imitation. Shakes a rattle, explores it with a finger and bangs on floor.

Plays 'peek-a-boo' and imitates hand-clapping.

Grasps toy in hand and offers to adult, but cannot yet give into adult's hand.

Watches toy being partially hidden under a cover or cup, and then finds it. May find toy wholly hidden under cushion or cup.

Only needs intermittent support when sitting on parent's or carer's lap and being dressed. When being carried by an adult, supports self in upright position and turns head to look around.

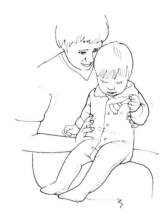

Grasps bell by handle and rings in imitation

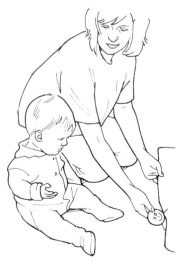

Watches while toy is partly hidden

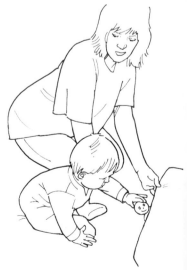

And promptly finds toy

Sits on floor for indefinite time. Can rise to sitting position from lying down.

Crawls on hands and knees, shuffles on buttocks or 'bear-walks' rapidly about the floor. May crawl upstairs.

Pulls to standing and sits down again, holding on to furniture. Walks around furniture lifting one foot and stepping sideways. Walks forward and sideways with one or both hands held. May stand alone for a few moments. May walk alone.

AGE 12 MONTHS

Posture and large movements

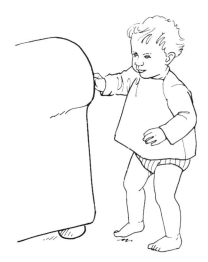

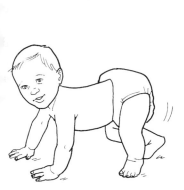

Bear-walks around floor

Steps sideways when holding on to settee

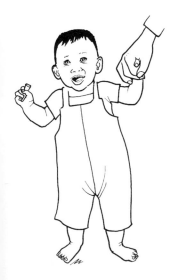

Walks with one hand held

AGE 12 MONTHS

Vision and fine movements

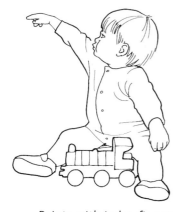

Points with index finger at object of interest

Picks up small objects with neat pincer grasp between thumb and tip of index finger.

Drops and throws toys forward deliberately and watches them fall to ground. Looks in correct place for toys which fall out of sight.

Points with index finger at objects of interest.

Out of doors, watches movement of people, animals or motor vehicles for prolonged periods. Recognises familiar people approaching from a distance.

Uses both hands freely but may show preference for one. Holds two toy bricks, one in each hand with tripod grasp, and bangs together to make noise.

Shows interest in pictures.

Hearing and speech

Knows and immediately responds to own name.

Babbles loudly and incessantly in conversational cadences. Vocalisation contains most vowels and many consonants. Shows by behaviour that words are understood in usual context, e.g. car, drink, cat. Understands simple instructions associated with a gesture, e.g. 'give it to Daddy', 'come to Mummy'.

Imitates adult playful vocalisations and may use a few words, with great enthusiasm.

May hand objects to adult on request or demonstrate understanding by use of objects, e.g. hair brush (definition-by-use)

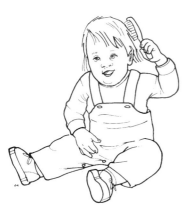

Definition-by-use of everyday objects

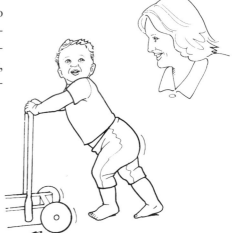

Immediately responds to own name

Drinks well from cup with little assistance. Holds spoon and will attempt to use for feeding, although very messy.

Helps with dressing by holding out arm for sleeve and foot for shoe.

Takes objects to mouth less often. Ceasing to drool.

Will put objects in and out of cup or box when shown.

Manipulates toys and will shake to make noise. Listens with pleasure to sound-making toys and repeats appropriate activity to reproduce sound. Gives toys to adults on request and sometimes spontaneously. Quickly finds toys hidden from view.

Likes to be in sight and hearing of familiar people. Demonstrates affection to familiars.

Plays 'pat-a-cake' and waves 'good-bye', both on request and spontaneously.

Sits, or sometimes stands, without support while dressed by carer.

AGE 12 MONTHS

Social behaviour and play

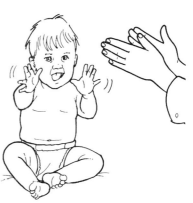

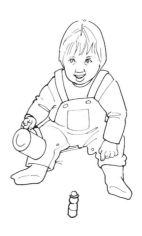

Plays 'pat-a-cake'

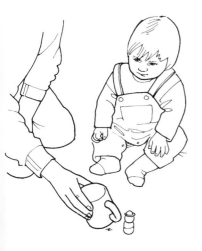

Watches while toy is hidden under cup

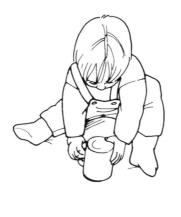

Regards and reaches for cup

Promptly finds toy

AGE 15 MONTHS

Posture and large movements

May walk alone, usually with uneven steps: feet wide apart, arms slightly flexed and held above head or at shoulder level for balance. Starts voluntarily, but frequently stopped by falling or bumping into furniture.

Lets self down from standing to sitting by collapsing backward with a bump, or by falling forward on hands and then back to sitting. Can get to feet alone.

Creeps upstairs safely, and may get downstairs backwards.

Kneels unaided or with support.

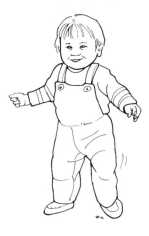

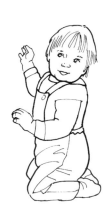

Walks alone, feet apart, arms assisting balance

Kneels unaided

Vision and fine movements

Picks up string or small objects with a precise pincer grasp, using either hand.

Manipulates cubes and may build a tower of two cubes after demonstration.

Grasps crayon with whole hand, using palmar grasp. Uses either hand, and imitates to and fro scribble.

Looks with interest at coloured pictures in book and pats page.

Watches small toy pulled across floor. Demands desired objects out of reach by pointing with index finger. Stands at window and watches outside happenings for several minutes, pointing to emphasise interest.

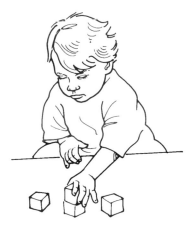

Manipulates cubes and builds tower of two

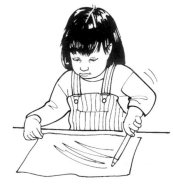

Grasps crayon with whole hand and scribbles to and fro

Hearing and speech

Makes many speech-like sounds. Says a few recognisable words (usually a range of between two to six) spontaneously in correct context, and demonstrates understanding of many more. Communicates wishes and needs by pointing and vocalising or screaming. Points to familiar persons, animals or toys when requested.

Understands and obeys simple instructions, such as 'don't touch', 'come for dinner', 'give me the ball'.

Social behaviour and play

Holds and drinks from a cup with the aid of an adult. Attempts to hold spoon, brings it to mouth and licks it, but is unlikely to prevent it turning over. Chews well.

Helps more constructively with dressing.

Pushes large, wheeled toy with handle on level ground.

Explores properties and possibilities of toys, convenient household objects and sound-makers with lively interest. Shows definition-by-use of common objects.

Carries dolls by limbs, hair or clothing. Repeatedly casts objects to floor in play or rejection, and watches where things fall. Looks for hidden toy.

Physically restless and intensely curious regarding people, objects and events.

Emotionally labile and closely dependent upon adult's reassuring presence. Is affectionate to familiar people.

Needs constant supervision for protection against dangers owing to extended exploration of the environment.

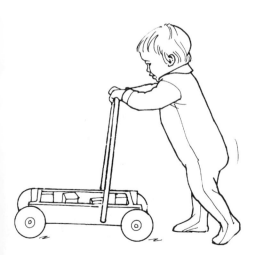

Pushes large, wheeled toy on level

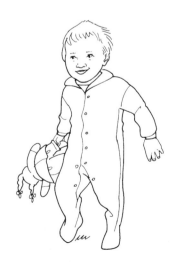

Carries doll by leg

AGE 18 MONTHS

Posture and large movements

Walks well with feet only slightly apart, starts and stops safely. No longer needs to hold upper arms in extension to balance.

Runs carefully, head held erect in midline, eyes fixed on ground one to two metres ahead, but finds difficulty in negotiating obstacles.

Pushes and pulls large toys or boxes along the floor.

Chooses to carry large doll or teddy-bear while walking. Backs into small chair or slides in sideways to seat self.

Enjoys climbing, and will climb forward into adult's chair, then turn round and sit.

Walks upstairs with helping hand and sometimes downstairs. Creeps backwards downstairs or occasionally bumps down a few steps on buttocks facing forwards.

Kneels upright on flat surface without support. Flexes knees and hips in squatting position to pick up toy from floor, and rises to feet using hands as support.

Note: Infants who 'bottom shuffle' are usually delayed in walking.

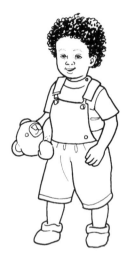

Walks well carrying toy

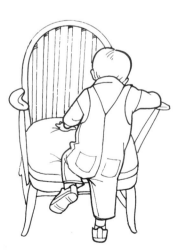

Climbs into adult chair

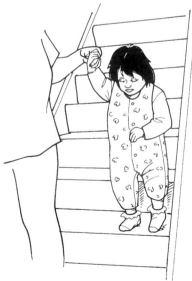

Walks up and down stairs with help

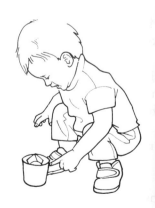

Squats to pick up fallen toy

*Vision and fine
movements*

cks up small objects immediately on sight with delicate pincer
asp.

Holds pencil in mid- or upper shaft in whole hand, or with
ude approximation of thumb and fingers. Spontaneous to and
o scribble and dots, using either hand alone or sometimes with
ncils in both hands.

Builds tower of three cubes after demonstration and sometimes
ontaneously.

Enjoys simple picture books, often recognising and putting
dex finger on boldly coloured items on page. Turns several pages
a time.

Beginning to show preference for using one hand.

Recognises familiar people at a distance and points to distant
teresting objects when outdoors.

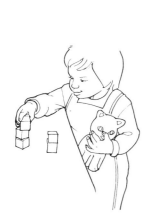 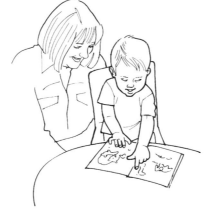

Builds tower of three cubes   Enjoys picture books

Hearing and speech

1akes speech-like sounds continually to self at play, with
onversational tunes and emotional inflections.

Listens and responds to spoken communications addressed
irectly to self. Uses between six and twenty recognisable words
nd understands many more. Echoes prominent or last word in
hort sentences addressed to self.

Demands a desired object by pointing accompanied by loud,
rgent vocalisations or single words.

Enjoys nursery rhymes and tries to join in. Attempts to sing.

Hands familiar objects to adult when requested. Obeys simple
nstructions, e.g. 'get your shoes' or 'shut the door'. Understands
10'. Points to own or doll's hair, shoes, nose, feet.

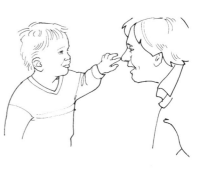

Points to person's nose

AGE 18 MONTHS

Social behaviour and play

Holds spoon and gets food safely to mouth, although may pl[a] with food. Holds cup between both hands and drinks witho[ut] much spilling. Lifts cup alone but usually hands back to adu[lt] when finished.

Assists with dressing and undressing, taking off shoes, sock[s] and hat, but seldom able to replace.

Beginning to give notice of urgent toilet needs by restlessne[ss] and vocalisation. Bowel control may be attained but very variab[le] May indicate wet or soiled pants.

Explores environment energetically and with increasing unde[r] standing. No sense of danger.

No longer takes toys to mouth.

Remembers where objects belong.

Still casts objects to floor in play or anger, but less often, an[d] seldom troubles visually to verify arrival on target.

Fascinated by household objects and imitates simple, everyda[y] activities such as feeding doll, reading book, brushing floo[r] washing clothes.

Plays contentedly alone but likes to be near familiar adult [or] older sibling. Emotionally still very dependent upon famili[ar] adult, alternating between clinging and resistance.

Enjoys putting small objects in and out of containers, an[d] learning the relative size of objects.

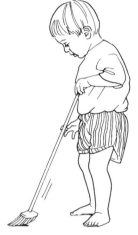

Imitates everyday activities

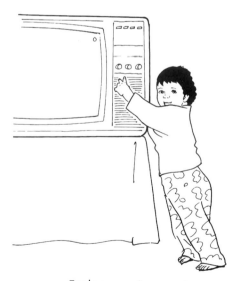

Explores environment

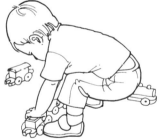

Plays contentedly alone

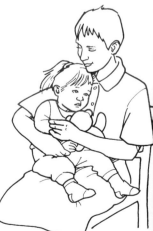

Still dependent upon familiar adult

uns safely on whole foot, stopping and starting with ease and
oiding obstacles.

Squats with complete steadiness to rest or to play with an
bject on the ground and rises to feet without using hands.

Pushes and pulls large, wheeled toys easily forwards and
ually able to walk backwards pulling handle. Pulls small
heeled toy by cord with obvious appreciation of direction.

Climbs on furniture to look out of window or to open doors
d can get down again.

Shows increasing understanding of size of self in relation to size
d position of objects in the environment, and to enclosed spaces
ch as a cupboard or cardboard box.

Walks upstairs and downstairs holding on to rail or wall; two
et to a step.

Throws small ball overhand and forwards, without falling over.
/alks into large ball when trying to kick it.

Sits on small tricycle, but cannot use pedals. Propels vehicle
rwards with feet on floor.

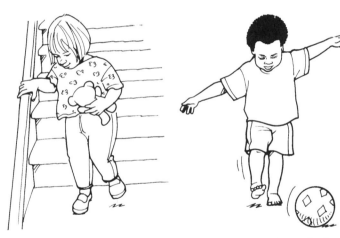

Walks up and down stairs   Walks into large ball

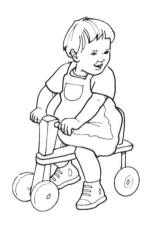

Sits and steers tricycle but cannot
yet use pedals

AGE 2 YEARS

Vision and fine movements

Good manipulative skills; picks up tiny objects accurately and quickly, and places down neatly with increasing skill.

Builds tower of six or seven cubes.

Holds a pencil well down shaft towards point, using thumb and first two fingers. Mostly uses preferred hand. Spontaneous circular scribble as well as to and fro scribble and dots; imitates vertical line and sometimes 'V' shape.

Enjoys picture books, recognising fine details in favourite pictures. Turns pages singly.

Recognises familiar adults in photograph after once shown, but not usually self as yet.

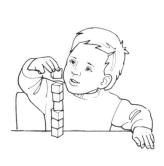

Builds tower of six or seven cubes

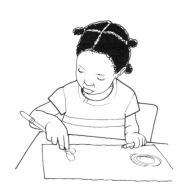

Holds pencil and scribbles

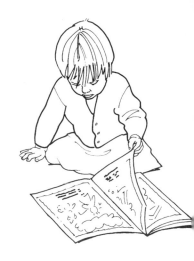

Enjoys books and turns pages singly

Uses fifty or more recognisable words appropriately and understands many more. Puts two or more words together to form simple sentences.

Attends to communications addressed to self and begins to listen with obvious interest to more general conversation. Refers to self by name and talks to self continually in long monologues during play, but may be incomprehensible to others.

Echolalia almost constant, with one or more stressed words repeated.

Constantly asking names of objects and people.

Joins in nursery rhymes and songs.

Indicates hair, hand, feet, nose, eyes, mouth, and shoes on request. Names familiar objects and pictures.

Carries out simple instructions such as 'go and see what the postman has brought'.

Beginning to show meaningful short sequence and definition-by-use of doll's house-sized toys.

AGE 2 YEARS

Hearing and speech

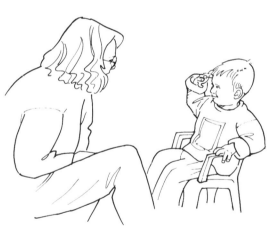

Points to hair on request

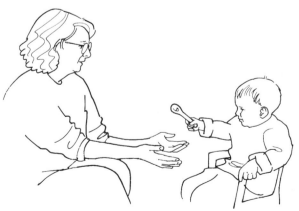

Hands familiar objects to adult

AGE 2 YEARS

Social behaviour and play

Feeds self competently with a spoon, but is easily distracted. Lifts cup and drinks well without spilling, and replaces cup on table without difficulty. Asks for food and drink.

Puts on hat and shoes.

Usually attempts to verbalise toilet needs in reasonable time, but still unreliable.

Intensely curious regarding environment. Turns door handles and often runs outside. Little comprehension of common dangers.

Follows parent or carer around house and imitates domestic activities in simultaneous play.

Spontaneously engages in simple role or situational make-believe activities.

Constantly demanding parent's or carer's attention. Clings tightly in affection, fatigue or fear, although resistive and rebellious when thwarted. Tantrums when frustrated or in trying to make self understood, but attention is usually readily distracted.

Defends own possessions with determination.

May take turns, but as yet has little idea of sharing either toys or the attention of adults.

Parallel play present; plays contentedly near other children but not with them.

Resentful of attention shown to other children, particularly by own familiars.

Unwilling to defer or modify immediate satisfaction of wishes.

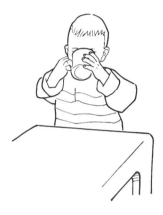

Lifts cup and drinks well without spilling

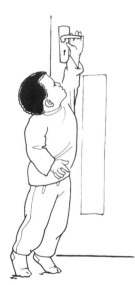

Turns door handles, has little comprehension of dangers

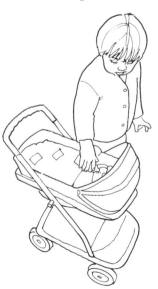

Engages in 'make-believe' play

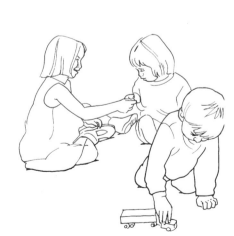

Plays near others but not with them

All locomotor skills rapidly improving. Walks upstairs confidently and downstairs holding rail, two feet to a step. Runs well and climbs easy nursery apparatus.

Pushes and pulls large toys skilfully but may have difficulty in steering them around obstacles.

Can jump with two feet together from a low step. Can stand on tiptoe if shown.

Throws ball from hand somewhat stiffly at body level. Kicks large ball, but gently and lopsidedly.

AGE 2½ YEARS

Posture and large movements

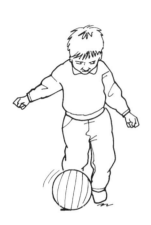

Kicks large ball gently

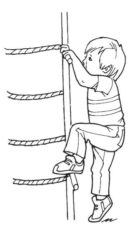

Climbs nursery apparatus

Builds tower of seven-plus cubes using preferred hand.

Recognises minute details in picture books.

Holds pencil in preferred hand, with improved tripod grasp. Imitates horizontal line and circle, and usually 'T' and 'V'.

Recognises self in photographs once shown.

Vision and fine movements

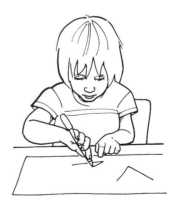

Holds pencil in preferred hand and copies 'V'

AGE 2½ YEARS

Hearing and speech

Uses two hundred or more recognisable words, but speech shows numerous immaturities of articulation and sentence structure. Knows full name. Talks audibly and intelligibly to self at play, concerning events happening here and now. Echolalia persists.

Continually asking questions beginning 'What?' or 'Who?'. Uses pronouns 'I', 'me' and 'you' correctly.

Stuttering in eagerness common. Says a few nursery rhymes. Enjoys simple familiar stories read from picture book.

Plays meaningfully with miniature doll's house-size toys, adding an intelligent, running commentary.

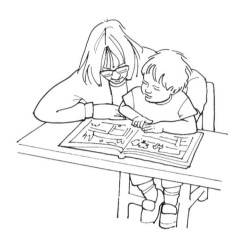

Enjoys picture books and stories

Social behaviour and play

Eats skilfully with spoon and may use a fork.

Pulls down pants when using the toilet, but seldom is able to replace them. May be dry through the night although this is extremely variable.

Exceedingly active, restless and resistive of restraint. Has little understanding of common dangers or need to defer immediate wishes.

Throws tantrums when thwarted and is less easily distracted. Emotionally still very dependent on adult.

More sustained role play, such as putting dolls to bed, washing clothes, driving motor cars, but with frequent reference to a friendly adult. Watches other children at play with interest, occasionally joining in for a few minutes, but as yet has little notion of the necessity to share playthings or adults' attention.

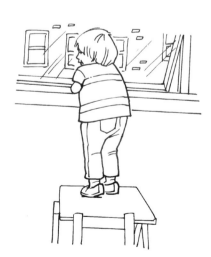

Active and curious with little notion of common dangers

Walks alone upstairs using alternating feet, comes downstairs two feet to a step, and can carry large toy. Usually jumps from bottom step with two feet together.

Climbs nursery apparatus with agility.

Can turn around obstacles and corners while running and also while pushing and pulling large toys. Walks forwards, backwards, sideways, etc., hauling large toys with complete confidence.

Obviously appreciates size and movements of own body in relation to external objects and space.

Rides tricycle using pedals, and can steer it round wide corners.

Can stand and walk on tiptoe. Can stand momentarily on one (preferred) foot when shown.

Can sit with feet crossed at ankles.

Can throw a ball overhand and catch large ball on or between extended arms. Kicks ball forcibly.

AGE 3 YEARS

Posture and large movements

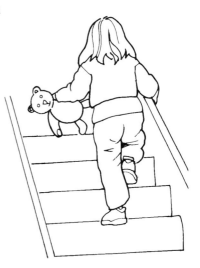

Walks upstairs and down carrying large toy

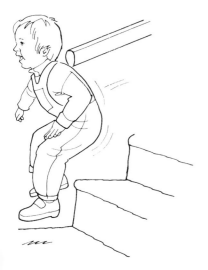

Jumps from bottom step (both feet together)

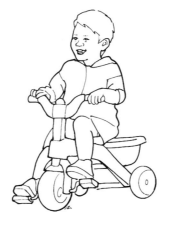

Rides tricycle using pedals

AGE 3 YEARS

Vision and fine movements

Builds tower of nine or ten cubes; by $3\frac{1}{2}$ years builds one or more bridges of three cubes from a model using two hands cooperatively. Threads large wooden beads on shoe lace.

Can close fist and wiggle thumb in imitation, right and left.

Holds pencil near the point in preferred hand, between the first two fingers and thumb, and uses it with good control. Copies circle, also letters 'V', 'H' and 'T'. Imitates a cross. Draws person with head and usually indication of one or two other features or parts.

Matches two or three primary colours; usually red and yellow, but may confuse blue and green. May know names of colours.

Enjoys painting with large brush on easel, covering whole paper with wash of colour or painting primitive 'pictures' which are usually named during or after production.

Cuts with toy scissors.

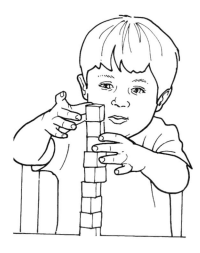

Builds tower of nine or ten cubes

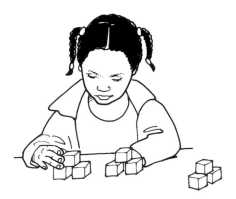

Builds several three-cube bridges
from a model

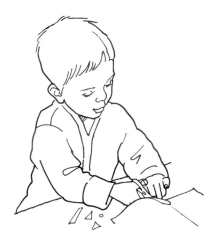

Cuts with scissors

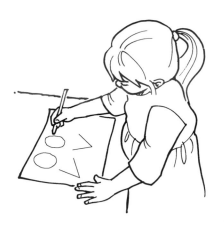

Copies circle and letter 'V'

Speech modulating in loudness and range of pitch. Large vocabulary intelligible even to strangers, but speech still contains many immature phonetic substitutions and unconventional grammatical forms.

Gives full name and sex, and sometimes age. Uses personal pronouns and plurals correctly and also most prepositions.

Still talks to self in long monologues, mostly concerned with the immediate present, particularly during make-believe activities. Carries on simple conversations and able to describe briefly present activities and past experiences.

Asks many questions beginning 'What?', 'Where? and 'Who?'.

Listens eagerly to stories and demands favourites over and over again. Knows several nursery rhymes to repeat and sometimes sing.

Counts by rote up to ten or more, but little appreciation of quantity beyond two or three.

AGE 3 YEARS

Hearing and speech

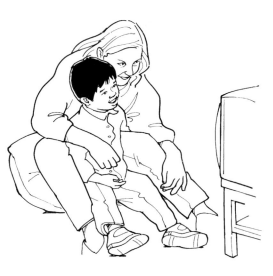

Enjoys watching television and will join in songs

AGE 3 YEARS

Social behaviour and play

Eats with a fork and spoon.

Washes hands but needs adult supervision with drying. Can pull pants down and up but needs help with buttons and other fastenings.

May be dry through the night, although this is very variable.

General behaviour is more amenable – can be affectionate and confiding.

Likes to help adults with domestic activities including gardening, shopping, etc.

Makes an effort to keep surroundings tidy.

Vividly realised make-believe play, including invented people and objects.

Enjoys playing on the floor with bricks, boxes, toy trains, dolls, prams, etc., alone or in company with siblings.

Joins in active make-believe play with other children. Understands sharing playthings.

Shows affection for younger siblings.

Shows some appreciation of difference between present and past and of the need to defer satisfaction of wishes to the future.

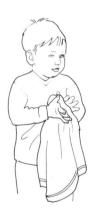

Washes hands but needs supervision with drying

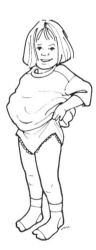

Can pull pants down and up

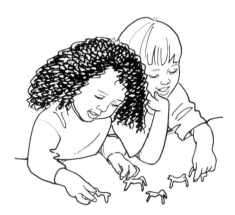

Joins in active make-believe play with other children

Walks or runs alone up and down stairs, one foot to a step in adult fashion. Navigates self-locomotion skilfully, turning sharp corners, running, pushing and pulling.

Climbs ladders and trees.

Can stand, walk and run on tiptoe.

Expert rider of tricycle, executing sharp 'U'-turns easily.

Stands on one (preferred) foot for three to five seconds and hops on preferred foot.

Arranges and picks up objects from floor by bending from waist with knees extended.

Sits with knees crossed.

Shows increasing skill in ball games, throwing, catching, bouncing, kicking, etc., including use of bat.

AGE 4 YEARS

Posture and large movements

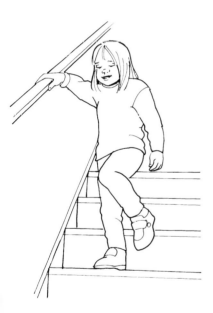

Walks up and down stairs in adult fashion

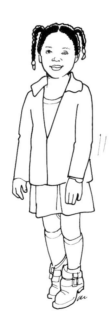

Stands and runs on tiptoe

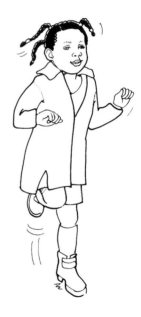

Hops on one foot

AGE 4 YEARS

Vision and fine movements

Builds tower of ten or more cubes and several bridges of three from one model on request or spontaneously. Builds three steps with six cubes after demonstration.

Imitates spreading of hand and bringing thumb into opposition with each finger in turn, right and left.

Holds and uses pencil with good control in adult fashion. Copies cross and also letters 'V', 'H', 'T' and 'O'. Draws a person with head, legs and trunk, and usually arms and fingers. Draws a recognisable house on request or spontaneously.

Beginning to name drawings before production.

Matches and names four primary colours correctly.

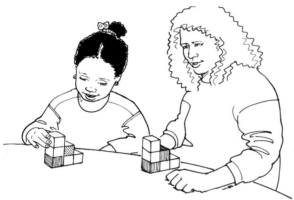

Builds three steps after demonstration

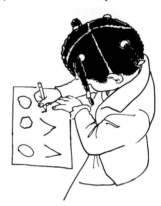

Copies circle and crosses

Hearing and speech

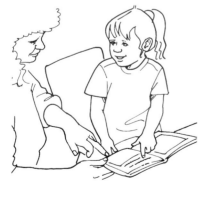

Enjoys listening to and telling stories

Speech grammatically correct and completely intelligible. Shows only a few immature phonetic substitutions, usually of r-l-w-y group, p-th-f-s group or k-t sound group. Gives connected account of recent events and experiences. Gives full name, home address and usually age.

Eternally asking questions 'Why?', 'When?', 'How?', and meanings of words.

Listens to and tells long stories, sometimes confusing fact and fantasy.

Counts by rote up to twenty or more, and beginning to count objects by word and touch in one-to-one correspondence up to four or five.

Enjoys jokes and verbal incongruities.

Knows several nursery rhymes which are repeated or sung correctly.

Eats skilfully with spoon and fork.

Washes and dries hands. Brushes teeth. Can undress and dress except for laces, ties and back buttons.

General behaviour more independent and strongly self-willed.

Inclined to verbal impertinence with adults and quarrelling with playmates when wishes crossed.

Shows sense of humour in talk and activities.

Dramatic make-believe play and dressing-up favoured. Floor games very complicated but habits less tidy.

Constructive out-of-doors building with any materials available.

Needs companionship of other children with whom he/she is alternately cooperative and aggressive, as with adults, but understands need to argue with words rather than blows. Understands taking turns as well as sharing.

Shows concern for younger siblings and sympathy for playmates in distress.

Appreciates past, present and future time.

AGE 4 YEARS

Social behaviour and play

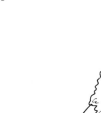

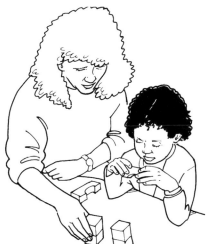

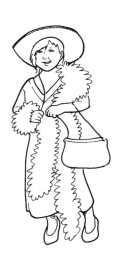

Dresses and undresses alone

Understands need for taking turns in play

Imaginative dressing-up play

AGE 5 YEARS

*Posture and large
movements*

Walks easily on narrow line. Runs lightly on toes. Active and skilful in climbing, sliding, swinging, digging and doing various 'stunts'. Skips on alternate feet.

Can stand on one foot eight to ten seconds, right or left, and usually also stands on preferred foot, with arms folded. Can hop two or three metres forwards on each foot separately.

Moves rhythmically to music.

Grips strongly with either hand.

Can bend and touch toes without flexing knees.

Plays all varieties of ball games with considerable ability, including those requiring appropriate placement or scoring, according to accepted rules.

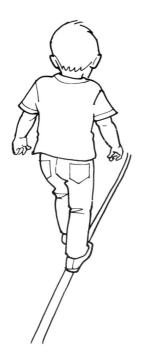

Walks on a narrow line

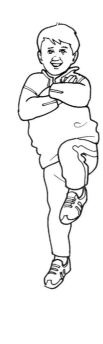

Stands on one foot with arms
folded

Picks up and replaces minute objects.

Builds elaborate models when shown, such as three steps with six cubes from model; sometimes four steps from ten cubes.

Good control in writing and drawing with pencils and paint brushes. Copies square and, at $5\frac{1}{2}$ years, a triangle. Also copies letters 'V', 'T', 'H', 'O', 'X', 'L', 'A', 'C', 'U' and 'Y'. Writes a few letters spontaneously.

Draws recognisable man with head, trunk, legs, arms and features. Draws house with door, windows, roof and chimney.

Spontaneously produces many other pictures containing several items and usually indication of background of environment, and names before production.

Colours pictures neatly, staying within outlines.

Counts fingers on one hand with index finger of other.

Names four or more primary colours and matches ten or twelve colours.

AGE 5 YEARS

Vision and fine movements

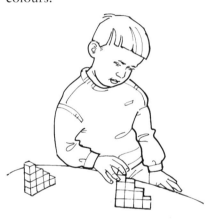
Constructs elaborate models

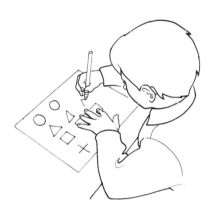
Copies squares and triangles

Speech fluent, grammatically conventional and usually phonetically correct except for confusions of s-f-th group. Delights in reciting or singing rhymes and jingles.

Loves to be read or told stories and acts them out in detail later, alone or with friends.

Gives full name, age and usually birthday. Gives home address.

Defines concrete nouns by use.

Constantly asks meaning of abstract words and uses them in and out of season.

Enjoys jokes and riddles.

Hearing and speech

AGE 5 YEARS

Social behaviour and play

Uses knife and fork competently.

Washes and dries face and hands but needs help or supervision for the rest. Undresses and dresses alone.

General behaviour more sensible, controlled and independent.

Comprehends need for order and tidiness, but needs constant reminder.

Domestic and dramatic play continued alone or with playmates from day to day.

Floor games very complicated.

Plans and builds constructively in and out of doors.

Chooses own friends. Cooperative with companions most of the time and understands need for rules and fair play.

Shows definite sense of humour.

Appreciates meaning of time in relation to daily programme.

Tender and protective towards younger children and pets. Comforts playmates in distress.

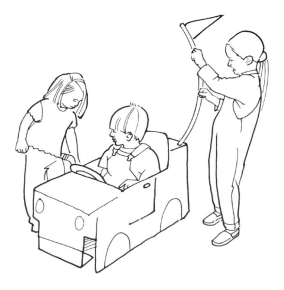

Engages in elaborate make-believe group play

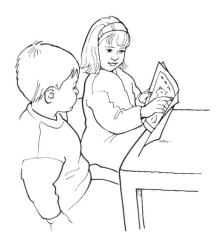

Affectionate and helpful to younger siblings

Bee, H., (1995), *The Developing Child* (7th edition), London, Harper-Collins.

Hall, D. (ed.), (1996), *Health for All Children* (3rd edition), Oxford, Oxford University Press.

Hall, D., Hill, P. and Elliman, D., (1996), *The Child Surveillance Handbook* (2nd edition), Oxford, Radcliffe Medical Press.

McMahon, L., (1995), *The Handbook of Play Therapy*, London, Routledge.

FURTHER READING

This section considers the patterns of development which are important for understanding developmental differences. While the majority of children follow a common pattern of development, variations sometimes occur that may or may not be significant. Details of the usual patterns of development in the areas of locomotor skills, vision, hearing, communication, language and speech are considered and suggestions made as to when it may be necessary to refer a child for specialist investigation. It is important that parental concerns are responded to appropriately, as parents are often the first to identify a problem. A brief explanation of testing procedures for checking vision and hearing is also included, although it is essential that these are carried out by trained personnel and that their limitations are recognised.

SECTION 2

Patterns of

Development

Posture and movement (locomotor skills)

Children's attainment of the ability both to move independently and to use their hands skilfully opens up the environment for them to explore, interact and learn. The development of these skills is helped by their interest and motivation and by playful interactions with carers.

The speed of development of motor progress is influenced by many factors and, while most children follow a fairly similar pattern, there is a wide variability in the age at which various skills may be achieved. Infants born very prematurely and nursed mainly on their backs may show early progress with supported standing, but be delayed in sitting unsupported. Lack of opportunities for infants to move freely, either because of being left in the cot, lack of stimulation or prolonged use of baby walkers, may delay developmental progress. Infants with severe visual impairment may also show a delay in acquiring locomotor skills. Children with excessively low muscle tone – floppiness (hypotonia) – or with high muscle tone – stiffness (hypertonia) – also show differences in the pattern and age of achievement of these skills.

Posture and large movements

Up to 90 per cent of infants will begin to sit independently at some time between six and eleven months, crawl between six and twelve months, walk alongside furniture from eight to thirteen months and achieve independent walking by the age of eighteen months (Capute *et al.* 1985). A small number of children may miss out the crawling stage and move from sitting independently to beginning to stand and walk. Between 10 and 15 per cent of children may follow a different pattern of achievement of these skills. They may prefer to move by rolling or bottom-shuffling before getting to stand and walk, which may be achieved as late as twenty to twenty-eight months. Such a child often has low muscle tone, and a similar history may be present in the family (Robson 1984).

Hand function (fine movements)

During the first year of life infants acquire the skill of approaching an object, first with both hands then with one hand, grasping objects with an increasingly refined grasp, transferring objects from one hand to the other, and releasing objects, first into containers and then with increasing precision building a tower of two toy bricks at about the age of twelve months. By three years of age, most children have acquired the ability to hold a pencil between the first two fingers and thumb using the preferred hand. There is a great deal of variability in the timing of establishing handedness, although most children establish it from the second year onwards. A strong preference for the use of one hand before the first birthday should indicate the need for further professional advice.

The variability in timing and pattern of achieving locomotor skills needs to be appreciated, and most children follow one of the known patterns. Although the majority of those who follow a less common pattern or are not walking by the age of eighteen months are likely to be normal (Chaplais and MacFarlane 1984), careful examination is required to rule out any problems.

When to seek advice

Vision

Development of visual behaviour

There is great variation in the visual behaviour of newborn infants depending on their level of alertness. When held in an upright position, newborn infants usually turn their eyes towards any large light source. The eye movements are not yet well coordinated; however, a constant squint occurring at any stage is abnormal.

During the first month of life infants stare at objects close to their face and show special interest in a human face, looking intensely into the eyes, particularly when they are being fed. They follow slow movement of the adult face through 90 degrees or more. A defensive blink is present from four to six weeks. At three months of age infants start watching the movements of their own hands and fingers and will follow activities in their surroundings. At six months, infants will look and fix on a 2.5 centimetre brick at 30 centimetres, and will regard it closely. They also look around with interest and recognise carers and familiar toys from across the room. By nine months they will look at, and use their fingers to poke, small objects up to 1 millimetre in size (e.g. crumbs or 'hundreds and thousands' cake decorations) at a distance of approximately 30 centimetres. Recognition of familiar adults from across the street also occurs at this time. By the age of one year infants point to demand objects, and, when outdoors, watch movements of people, animals, cars, etc., with prolonged and intense regard.

Assessment of visual problems in young children

Many of the conditions which lead to severe visual impairment, such as congenital cataract, retinopathy of prematurity, glaucoma and retinoblastoma, are treatable if detected early. A careful inspection of the eyes is a mandatory part of newborn examination. An ophthalmoscope should be used with a +3 lens from a distance of 20–25 centimetres to look for the red reflex. The inspection and examination should be repeated at six to eight weeks. Parental concerns can identify many early and serious visual problems and the use of a parental checklist can be helpful (see Appendix 2). Parents should be asked, soon after the birth and at any subsequent visit, whether they have any concerns about the baby's vision. Specialist examination is required for known high-risk groups, including low-birth weight infants at risk of retinopathy of prematurity, babies with a close family history of potentially heritable eye disorder, and children with dysmorphic syndromes or neurodevelopmental problems (Hall 1996).

Assessment of visual behaviour

Abnormalities of visual behaviour for children under the age of three years, such as poor visual fixation and following and wandering eye movements, may indicate the presence of a visual defect. Tests of visual behaviour, including the observation of sharp fixation for sweets of 1 millimetre diameter at a distance of 30 centimetres, only exclude serious visual problems and do not offer any measurement of visual acuity (Sonksen 1993).

Formal tests for visual acuity in children under the age of three years are best carried out by an orthoptist or a trained person, owing to the problems of cooperation and understanding of the test. Methods of forced choice preferential looking, visual-evoked responses and optokinetic nystagmus are used for specialist assessment. From the age of three years, visual acuity for distance vision can be assessed using picture tests (e.g. Kay, Elliot) or letter charts with matching cards or letters. A Snellen-type chart is preferable to single letters (Stycar tests or Sheridan Gardener cards) because the latter may seriously underestimate or miss the diagnosis of amblyopia (Hilton and Stanley 1972). Each eye must be tested separately, with the other eye occluded. The Sonksen–Silver test of visual acuity is validated for use at 3 metres distance.

Assessment of visual acuity

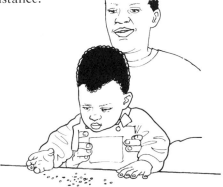

Looks sharply at small objects up to 1 millimetre in size at a distance of approximately 30 centimetres (age 8 months)

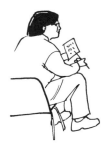
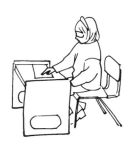

Visual acuity testing using Sonksen–Silver test (for age 3 years onwards)

Detection of squint

The presence of squint may indicate poor visual acuity and may predispose to amblyopia and impaired binocular vision. The majority of manifest squints are first recognised by parents, and they should always be asked whether they have noticed any squint, laziness or turning of one eye. Some squints are not noticeable on simple inspection and the corneal reflection test (observing the symmetry of reflection in both eyes), the cover–uncover test or the alternate cover test may be used. The performance and interpretation of these methods is not easy, and orthoptic assessment should be arranged in case of doubt and the presence of parental concern or relevant family history.

Further reading

Hyvarinen, L., (1988), *Vision in Children: Normal and Abnormal*, Ontario, The Canadian Deaf–Blind and Rubella Association.

Sonksen, P. M. and Stiff, B., (1991), *Show Me What My Friends Can See: A Developmental Guide for Parents of Babies with Severely Impaired Sight and their Professional Advisors*, London, The Wolfson Centre.

Newborn infants often respond to loud sounds by startle reflex or stilling. Their eyes may reflexly turn towards the direction of the sound. By one month of age they pause to listen and may turn their eyes and head to sounds. By the age of four months infants consistently turn towards sounds.

Over the next six months their attempt to locate the sound matures, head and neck control improves and the ability to sit is developed. By the age of six or seven months they turn immediately towards the parent's or carer's voice and visually engage. By the age of nine months they begin to search for very quiet sounds made out of sight and make precise attempts to locate them. At this stage an infant is able to distinguish meaningful sounds, such as the parent's or carer's voice.

Infants with an impairment of hearing, or those brought up in a noisy environment, may fail to develop interest and ability in hearing, and this failure often raises parental concerns. The use of a parental checklist (see Appendix 1) helps to alert parents to the existence of hearing loss. It is important that parents are asked whether they have any concerns regarding their child's hearing, and if there is any family history of hearing problems. Parents are more likely to identify severe and profound hearing loss, and may easily overlook less severe or high-frequency impairments.

Since most cases of significant sensorineural hearing loss are congenital, various technological approaches have been developed for assessing the hearing of infants. At this stage, brainstem-evoked response audiometry and evoked otoacoustic emissions are the most promising methods.

The distraction test depends on the infant's ability to turn and localise a sound source. A developmental level of around seven months is optimum for this test. Beyond ten months of age, the development of object permanence and increasing sociability make this test more difficult.

Two *trained* personnel, working in collaboration, are required to perform the test. Quiet conditions, proper equipment, adequate sound level monitoring and careful technique are all essential. One person, the distractor, works in front of the infant to hold the infant's attention using toys, etc. When the infant is distracted towards the toy the distractor hides the toy and the second person presents the test stimulus from behind the child. The sound source should be located at a level horizontal with the infant's ear, at a distance of approximately one metre from the ear and outside the infant's field of vision (or at a specified distance if warblers are

Hearing

Development of hearing

Age-appropriate tests of hearing
Neonatal screening

Behavioural testing during the first year of life

The distraction test

used). The distractor observes the infant's response. The definite response is a full 90-degree head turn towards the sound source. Any other outcome is an indication to re-test in four to six weeks, or to refer immediately if the parents are concerned or there are special circumstances.

For screening purposes the sounds are produced at minimal levels (< 35 dB). High and low frequencies are tested separately. A special Manchester rattle (or Nuffield rattle), the consonant 's' repeated rhythmically for high frequencies and an unmodified voice 'hum' or rhythmical repetition of a nursery rhyme (low frequency) are used. Whispering or quiet speaking is not acceptable. Frequency-modulated 'warble' tones are used to test a range of frequencies.

When inadequately performed, this test can be harmful by delaying identification of problems or by generating a large number of false positive referrals. Good results can be obtained if initial and regular refresher training is provided to the testers to ensure meticulous technique.

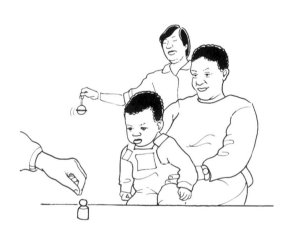

Distracting the infant with a toy

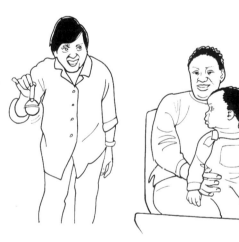

Using Manchester rattle at ear level, infant turns head 90 degrees to sound source

These tests rely upon the child's ability to respond to simple requests. Traditionally, this has involved asking the child to point to parts of the body or to follow simple requests like 'give it to Mummy', without any visual clues. From the age of two years onwards, speech discrimination tests like the *McCormick Toy Test* can be performed. The test has fourteen words in seven pairs, and a child with normal hearing should identify at least 80 per cent of the items at a voice level of 40 dB (McCormick 1993). An automated version of the test is now available.

Note: It is important to be aware that a child may fail a speech discrimination test either because of hearing difficulty or because of delayed language development.

Cooperation tests for 18–30 months of age

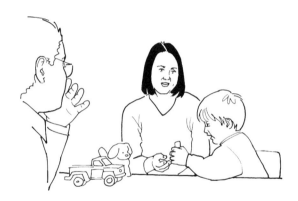

Child responds to request 'give the toy to Mummy'

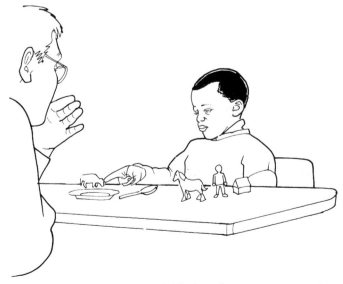

McCormick Toy Test – child identifies toy on request

Performance testing for over 30 months of age

These tests depend upon the child's ability to make an unambiguous response (e.g. putting 'a man in a boat' or 'bricks in a box') on production of a sound at different frequencies, either with a hand-held audiometer or with headphones (*pure tone audiometry*). The test can also be performed using the voice. The sounds 'go' (low frequency) and 'ss' (high frequency) can be used to prompt the required response from the child. The voice should be lowered to 40 dB and visual clues avoided by covering the mouth.

Further reading

McCormick, B., (1988), *Screening for Hearing Impairment in Young Children*, Beckenham, Croom Helm.

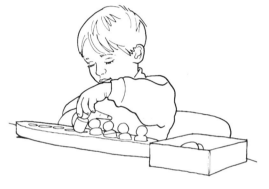

Child responds to prompt 'go' or 'ss' by putting 'man in a boat'

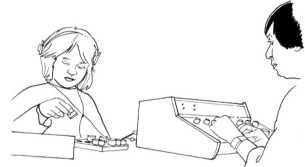

Pure tone audiometry

A child who is slow to talk often raises parental and professional concern. However, there are wide variations among normal children in the rate of language acquisition. The child's social interaction skills and the ability to understand language need to be considered to define the nature of the problem.

Early interactions between infants and parents are mainly exchanges of emotions, and start soon after birth with eye contact and changes in the infant's behavioural state (Brazelton 1995). As these responses become more complex, reciprocal interactions around caregiving and play activities emerge so that, by six to eight weeks, an infant smiles in response to a social interaction, giving great pleasure to carers. From three to six months, infants show their preference for an object by sustained looking. They show readiness for interaction by turning and looking in an interested manner with varying facial expressions. By eight to ten months, infants can coordinate their interest in objects and people by gaining carers' attention and looking at or grasping an object at the same time. Gestures are increasingly used in combination with vocalisation to demand objects and to share feelings about objects and events. Pointing with the index finger is one of the most important communicative gestures to develop, as it draws others into interaction with the child and also elicits naming (Bates *et al.* 1979); it begins to be seen from nine months and, by eighteen months, infants point to objects to express their interest and to share this interest with others. They are able to follow when an object is pointed out to them. Carers can help to establish communication by looking at and pointing to objects and naming them.

How much a child understands can be difficult to establish. Early communication takes place in familiar situations where routines and daily experiences help children to make good guesses with little need for actual understanding of what is being said.

There is enormous diversity in the way that children develop their early understanding of language. This reflects both the contribution of the individual child and also the variety of games and social interactions in which different families engage. From six to nine months an infant may recognise one or two words for objects, such as 'tick-tock' for clock, or may show an appropriate response to 'bye-bye' or 'clap hands'. From now onwards the infant begins to show an understanding of frequently repeated

Communication, language and speech

Early communication
Establishing interaction

Understanding of language

words and short sentences when used in familiar situations, assisted greatly by gestures and actions. By their first birthday, most children will recognise some everyday objects without the help of gestural clues (Fletcher 1987).

During their second year, children will recognise new words at an ever-increasing rate and understand up to two key words in familiar commands (Bates *et al.* 1995). During their third year they will understand prepositions of increasing complexity (in, on, under), action words (eating, running), and will begin to understand size differences (little doll). From the age of three years, children develop their understanding of colour, position and negatives; they understand pretend situations and increasingly use language for thought and reasoning. By the age of five, children understand long and complex sentences and such concepts as 'what happens next?'.

Expressive language
Babble, pre-words and the first few words

At six to eight weeks an infant produces the first comfort or 'cooing' sounds. These sounds soon diversify to contain a range of vowels and some consonants. At about four months of age laughter-like sounds emerge. Babbling becomes increasingly complex, and towards the end of the first year strings of syllables like 'mamama' or 'papapa' are produced. From about ten to fourteen months, infants may produce word-like sounds – 'pre-words' (dis, na, da) – to convey approval, disapproval, request or rejection. Gestures are often used with these sounds to add meaning. The age at which the first recognisable word is spoken is highly variable, even within the same family. By the first birthday most children are using a combination of tuneful babble and pre-words, while some also have a few recognisable words. Gradually the babble, pre-words and gestures are added to and then replaced by an expanding recognisable spoken vocabulary (Halliday 1975).

Word combinations and grammar

Although most children will combine two words together by the age of two years, up to 10 per cent will master this during the third year of life (Bates *et al.* 1995). Within the next few months children will use simple three-element sentences ('Mummy see me'). In the next stage children begin to develop grammatical systems, simple clause structure and the use of interrogatives. All children initially make certain 'errors' to simplify the task, such as using past tense constructions such as 'comed' and 'goed', which persist for quite some time before being gradually dropped. By the age of four years a child may be able to retell a simple story using coordinate clauses ('After we finished our dinner, we went outside and played a game'). From this stage onwards a child is able to hold simple conversations which gradually increase in complexity.

In the early stages of using single words, children may only use a limited set of sounds. As their vocabulary increases during the later part of the second and the early part of the third year, children seem to simplify the task by using different strategies. They may miss out the first or the final consonant (ish for fish), replace the first with the final consonant and sometimes add an extra vowel at the end (gogi for dog), replace certain sounds (tea for sea, tup for cup) or reduce words (pam for pram). They will modulate the tone of their speech sounds to express emotional meaning, to emphasise or to question. By four years of age most children are intelligible to strangers, although certain immaturities may persist well into primary school.

Between the ages of two and nine years, when children are learning to talk at a rapid rate, many children, often when excited or angry, have mild features of dysfluency (stammering). This usually takes the form of repetition of sounds (M-M-M-Mummy), syllables (Mum-Mum-Mum-Mummy) and words (what-what-what). Like other speech skills, fluency gradually improves with age. Preventive specialist advice is needed if there is parental concern, a history of stammering in the family, or the child shows signs of tension while struggling to speak.

Attention is children's ability to look, listen and concentrate on what they see or hear, and is an area in which many language-delayed children are immature (Cooper *et al.* 1978), although attention depends to some extent on the situation and on the nature of the task.

Children are extremely open to distraction during the first year of life as their attention is held momentarily by whatever is interesting in the environment. During the second year, children rigidly attend to their own choice of activity, particularly when the rewards are immediate and are part of the activity. They do not like external directions and interruptions. During the third year, children are usually able to interrupt a task to receive directions. Before any directions are given, their attention must be fully focused, and help may be needed in relating them to the task. Most children begin to control their attention from the age of four years, and are able to listen to any directions without interrupting the task.

Speech and fluency

Attention control

The great diversity, and when to ask for advice

Children show a great variation in the development of language skills which is often apparent even between two children in the same family. Although failure to talk is the most obvious cause of concern, the child's ability to interact, to use gestures, to imagine or pretend and to understand language are more significant indicators of a child's normalcy or need for help. The age norms given above are averages, and can only serve as a guide to the way language skills usually develop. However, any delay or unusual features can be the first indication of a problem for which a child may need help.

Note: Hearing problems can adversely affect children's speech and language, and it is important to get a child's hearing tested if there are any concerns.

Further reading

Byrne, R., (1991), *Let's Talk About Stammering* (revised edition), London, The Association for Stammerers.

Cooper, J., Moodley, M. and Reynell, J., (1978), *Helping Language Development*, London, Edward Arnold.

Law, J. and Elias, J., (1996), *Trouble Talking: A Guide for Parents of Children with Speech and Language Difficulties*, London, Jessica Kingsley Publishers.

Richman, N. and Lansdown, R., (1988), *Problems of Pre-School Children*, Chichester, Wiley.

The following checklists can be used by parents to help them to identify the patterns of development associated with hearing and vision development, and to help them to access the appropriate support services if their child has special needs.

APPENDIX 1 CHECKLIST FOR DETECTION OF HEARING PROBLEM

Hint for parents

Can your baby hear you?

Here is a checklist of some of the general signs you can look for in your baby's first year (with acknowledgements to Dr Barry McCormick). Does your baby display the following characteristics?

YES/NO

Shortly after birth
Your baby should be startled by a sudden loud noise such as a hand clap or a door slamming, and should blink or open her/his eyes widely to such sounds.

By 1 month
Your baby should be beginning to notice sudden or prolonged sounds like the noise of a vacuum cleaner and s/he should pause and listen to them when they begin.

By 4 months
S/he should quieten or smile at the sound of your voice when s/he cannot see you. S/he may also turn her/his head or eyes towards you if you come up from behind and speak to her/him from the side.

By 7 months
S/he should turn immediately to your voice from across the room or to very quiet noises on each side if s/he is not too occupied with other things.

By 9 months
S/he should listen attentively to familiar everyday sounds and search for very quiet sounds made out of sight. S/he should also show pleasure in babbling loudly and tunefully.

By 12 months
S/he should show some response to her/his own name and to other familiar words. S/he may also respond when you say 'no' and 'bye-bye', even when s/he cannot see any accompanying gesture.

> Your health visitor will perform a routine hearing test on your baby between six and eight months of age. She will be able to help and advise you at any time before or after this test if you are concerned about your baby and her/his development. If you suspect that your baby is not hearing normally, either because you cannot answer 'yes' to the items above or for some other reason, seek advice from your health visitor.

© Dr Barry McCormick, Children's Hearing Assessment Centre, Nottingham

APPENDIX 2 CHECKLIST FOR DETECTION OF VISION PROBLEM

Here are some of the signs of normal vision for you to look out for during your baby's first year:

From 1 week
- Does your baby turn to diffuse light?
- Does your baby stare at your face?

By 2 months
- Does your baby look at you, follow your face if you move from side to side, and smile responsively back at you?
- Do your baby's eyes move together?

By 6 months
- Does your baby look around with interest?
- Does your baby try to reach out for small objects?
- Do you think your baby has a squint? Squint is now definitely abnormal, however slight and temporary.

By 9 months
- Does your baby poke and rake very small objects such as crumbs or 'hundreds and thousands' cake decorations with fingers?

By 12 months
- Does your baby point to things to demand?
- Does your baby recognise people s/he knows from across the room, before they speak to her/him?

If at any time you suspect that your baby's vision is not normal, either because you cannot answer 'yes' to any of the items above or you suspect a squint, seek advice from your health visitor or general practitioner.

APPENDIX 3 CHECKLIST OF SUPPORT SERVICES FOR CHILDREN WITH SPECIAL NEEDS

(adapted from HVA Special Interest Group for CSN checklist)

Birth onwards
• Do you require information about local or nationwide support organisations or resources?
• Do you want to be put in contact with another family in a similar situation?
• Is your child likely to need specialist daycare?
• Will you require help from such schemes as Respite Care, Crossroads, etc.?
• Could you and your child benefit from Portage?
• Is your child's name on the Social Services Disability Register (Children Act 1989)?
• Are you eligible for financial help from the Family Fund?
• Is your child attending medical checks and routine surveillance?
• Have you received genetic counselling if appropriate?

Age 3 months onwards
• Are you eligible for Disability Living Allowance or Invalid Care Allowance?
• Has dental care for your child been discussed and a suitable dentist accessed?

Rising 2 years
• Has the Education Department been informed of your child's special needs?
• Do you need an orange badge/sticker for your car to facilitate parking?

Age 2 to 5 years (and beyond)
• Do you require information about Special Education Statementing and Code of Practice?

Age 3 years (may vary)
• Is your child eligible for disposable nappies/incontinence pads, etc.?

Rising 5 years
Are you entitled to:
• Disability Living Allowance (mobility component)?
• Motability?
• Vehicle Excise Duty (car tax) exemption?

If you require further information or advice about any of the above services, please contact your CDT, health visitor, general practitioner or social worker.

Bates, E., Benigni, L., Bretherton, I., Camaioni, I. and Volterra, V., (1979), *The Emergence of Symbols: Communication and Cognition in Infancy*, New York, Academic Press.

Bates, E., Dal, P. S. and Thal, D., (1995), 'Individual Differences and Their Implications for Theories of Language Development', in P. Fletcher and B. MacWhinney (eds), *The Handbook of Child Language*, London, Blackwell.

Bee, H., (1995), *The Developing Child* (7th edition), London, Harper-Collins.

Brazelton, T. B., (1995), *Neonatal Behaviour Assessment Scale No. 137*, Cambridge, Cambridge University Press.

Byrne, R., (1991), *Let's Talk About Stammering* (revised edition), London, The Association for Stammerers.

Capute, A. J., Shapiro, B. K., Palmer, F. B., Ross, A. and Wachtel, R. C., (1985), 'Normal Gross Motor Development: The Influences of Race, Sex and Socio-economic Status', *Developmental Medicine and Child Neurology*, 27, 635–643.

Chaplais, de Z. J. and MacFarlane, J. A., (1984), 'A Review of 404 Late Walkers', *Archives of Diseases in Childhood*, 59, 512–516.

Cooper, J., Moodley, M. and Reynell, J., (1978), *Helping Language Development*, London, Edward Arnold.

Department for Education, (1994), *Code of Practice on the Identification and Assessment of Special Educational Needs*, London, Central Office of Information.

Fletcher, P. (1987), 'Aspects of Language Development in the Preschool Years', in W. Yule and M. Rutter (eds), *Language Development and Disorders, No. 101/102*, Cambridge, Cambridge University Press.

Hall, D. (ed.), (1996), *Health for All Children* (3rd edition), Oxford, Oxford University Press.

Hall, D., Hill, P. and Elliman, D., (1996), *The Child Surveillance Handbook* (2nd edition), Oxford, Radcliffe Medical Press.

Halliday, M., (1975), *Learning How to Mean: Exploration in the Development of Language*, London, Edward Arnold.

Hilton, A. F. and Stanley, J. C., (1972), 'Pitfalls in Testing Children's Vision by the Sheridan Gardiner Single Optotype Method', *British Journal of Ophthalmology*, 56, 135–138.

Hyvarinen, L., (1988), *Vision in Children: Normal and Abnormal*, Ontario, The Canadian Deaf–Blind and Rubella Association.

Illingworth, R., (1992), *The Development of the Infant and Young Child* (9th edition), London, Churchill Livingstone.

Kimpton, D., (1990), *A Special Child in the Family*, London, Sheldon Press.

Law, J. and Elias, J., (1996), *Trouble Talking: A Guide for Parents of Children with Speech and Language Difficulties*, London, Jessica Kingsley Publishers.

McCormick, B., (1988), *Screening for Hearing Impairment in Young Children*, Beckenham, Croom Helm.

—— (1993), *Paediatric Audiology 0–5 Years* (2nd edition), London, Whurr Publishers.

McMahon, L., (1995), *The Handbook of Play Therapy*, London, Routledge.

NHS Executive, (1996), *Child Health in the Community*, London, Department of Health.

Polnay, L. (Chair of Joint Working Party), (1995), *Health Needs of School Age Children*, London, British Paediatric Association.

Prechtl, H. F. R., (1977), *The Neurological Examination of the Full Term Newborn Infant* (2nd edition), Clinics in Developmental Medicine No. 63, London: Heinemann.

Richman, N. and Lansdown, R., (1988), *Problems of Pre-School Children*, Chichester, Wiley.

Robson, P., (1984), 'Pre-walking Locomotor Movements and Their Use in Predicting Standing and Walking', *Child Care Health and Development*, 10, 317.

SCOPE (formerly the Spastics Society), (1994), *Right from the Start*, London, SCOPE.

Sheridan, M. D., (1975), *From Birth to Five Years*, Windsor, NFER-Nelson.

Sonksen, P. M., (1993), 'The assessment of Vision in the Pre-school Child', *Archives of Diseases in Childhood*, 68, 513–516.

Sonksen, P. M. and Stiff, B., (1991), *Show Me Ehat My Friends Can See: A Developmental Guide for Parents of Babies with Severely Impaired Sight and Their Professional Advisors*, London, The Wolfson Centre.

Yerbury, M. and Thomas, J., (1994), 'Health Visitors' Role in Services for Children with Disabilities', *Health Visitor*, 3, 67, 86–87.